A Better Normal for Pain

Your Guide to Rediscovering Intimacy After
Cancer

Tess Devèze

Published in Australia by ConnectAble Therapies Pty Ltd.

1510 Mills Road, Glen Forrest WA 6071, Australia
Copyright © 2023 Tess Devèze
All rights reserved.

Disclaimer: All care has been taken in the preparation of the information herein, but no responsibility can be accepted by the author for any damages resulting from the misinterpretation of this work. The content in this book shall not be used as an alternative to seeking professional and clinical advice.

For more information see www.connectabletherapies.com

ISBN: 978-0-6458244-8-3

CONTENTS

WHY I WROTE THIS BOOK

Hello! It's so wonderful to meet you. I'm Tess.

I thought before we get into the more 'intimate' details, I'd introduce myself and let you know what this book is about.

I was diagnosed with stage-three breast cancer in 2018, at the age of 36. At the time of my diagnosis, I'd been working in the sexuality sector for years. Over the years since my cancer diagnosis and endless treatments, only twice did a healthcare professional voluntarily bring up the topic of sexuality and only one booklet was recommended to me (which I had to go and find myself). The lack of information and support on this topic, both during and after treatments, was painfully noticeable.

Why aren't more resources available? Why are we so afraid to talk about this essential aspect of our lives?

First and foremost, I'm an occupational therapist (OT). What's an OT, I hear you ask? We are functional therapists and use specific approaches to promote independence and participation in 'occupations' which are any kind of meaningful life activity that occupies us. OT's help you do the day-to-day activities that you need and want to do, as best you can. This may include self-care tasks (shower, dressing, toileting), work related (vocational) tasks, social or community activities…and may also include sex!

My clinical experience is mostly in sexuality - during and after cancer treatments, brain-injury, neurological conditions, and those living with disability. Before moving solely to sexuality for people with cancer, disability and chronic illness, most of my work was in private and public hospitals across Australia, working in neurological rehabilitation. I love neuroscience, and most of my work is based on neurological concepts.

Other than having cancer and being a sexuality OT, I also work with sexuality and self-development pioneers 'Curious Creatures', based in Melbourne Australia. I've facilitated hundreds of workshops online and face to face for nearing a decade, teaching consent, better intimacy and communication skills. I've seen thousands of people's lives change through a deeper understanding of sexual intimacy.

Lastly, I've also studied somatic sexological bodywork at the Institute of Somatic Sexology. This training has given me a deeper understanding of how libido, pleasure, arousal and orgasmicity (cool word huh?) work on a physiological, neurological, and psychological level. These learnings form an essential part of this book.

Even with all my training, I've struggled. If you're struggling too, you're not alone (even if it doesn't get spoken about).

But it's not just about me. The contents of this book are also guided by you. I have a Facebook group 'Intimacy and Cancer' with thousands of people - all cancers, all genders - from over 49 countries, who share and support each other on this topic. My one-on-one clients have also been a huge source of learning, generously sharing their experiences.

It's been almost two years since releasing 'A Better Normal; Your Guide to Rediscovering Intimacy After Cancer', and the positive feedback I have personally been receiving from readers has been at times overwhelming. I am humbled, amazed and inspired by the impact and influence this book has had for those out there suffering.

But cancer treatments are *haaaaaard*, and so is reading! I wanted to know how I could reach more people, change more lives for the better through the contents in this book. In answer to that question, I've created the 'A Better Normal' mini-book *series*. It's a number of bite-sized treatment or side-effect specific mini-books, to help cancer patients and their loved ones maintain and grow connection, intimacy and sexuality. Each mini-book is created from the information in 'A Better Normal; Your Guide to Rediscovering Intimacy After Cancer', but broken down into simple, easy-to-read guides relative to your very specific needs, because often during and after treatments committing to a 300-page book feels overwhelming or is simply not possible.

Books in the 'A Better Normal' mini-book series are:

- 'A Better Normal for **Libido**; Your Guide to Rediscovering Intimacy After Cancer'
- 'A Better Normal for **Vaginal Dryness & Pain**; Your Guide to Rediscovering Intimacy After Cancer'
- 'A Better Normal for **Body Confidence**; Your Guide to Rediscovering Intimacy After Cancer'
- 'A Better Normal for **Chemotherapy**; Your Guide to Rediscovering Intimacy After Cancer'
- 'A Better Normal for **Hormone Therapy**; Your Guide to Rediscovering Intimacy After Cancer'
- 'A Better Normal for **Fatigue**; Your Guide to Rediscovering Intimacy After Cancer'

- 'A Better Normal for **Changes In Erection**; Your Guide to Rediscovering Intimacy After Cancer'
- 'A Better Normal for **Radiotherapy**; Your Guide to Rediscovering Intimacy After Cancer'
- 'A Better Normal for **Pain**; Your Guide to Rediscovering Intimacy After Cancer'

Or if you're after all of the above information (and more) in one place, the all-in-one book 'A Better Normal; Your Guide to Rediscovering Intimacy After Cancer' has everything you need.

If you end up with several mini-books in the series, that's pretty normal, as we don't have only one side-effect (geez, wouldn't that be nice!), and we can have the same side-effect from more than one treatment (like fatigue, or changes in libido). Cancer treatments impact us differently, which is why some books in this series are side-effect specific, and others treatment specific. So you can pick and choose what is most relevant for you and where you're at. You'll also notice that some mini-books have repeated information in them. That's because some information is essential and helpful, regardless of what your side-effect or treatment is (like the communication tips, or ways to gently reconnect with yourself or a partner).

The most important thing you can learn from this book is that you're not alone and you're not broken. There's nothing wrong with you if you're struggling. It's normal to find this situation tough. This isn't one-size-fits-all advice. All bodies are unique, every relationship is different, and everyone experiences relationships, connection, pleasure and desire in their own way. You're the expert on you! Just as cancer is different for everyone, so are the connections we have with ourselves and those around us.

Lastly, this book is for all human beings, regardless of gender, lifestyle, orientation, ability, ethnicity, age, or relationship dynamic. Although every person with cancer is unique, we have one thing in common: no matter who we are or what we are going through, we're all worthy of love and connection.

Now, let's get started on making your 'new normal', a 'better normal'.

1. KEY TERMS EXPLAINED

Sexuality vs sex

The word 'sexuality' is an umbrella term which yes includes the functional activity of sex, but also includes relationships, connections, affection, dating, pleasure and our overall well-being. Sexuality can be greatly affected due to cancer, but it doesn't necessarily have to stop altogether. As a sexuality educator and clinician, I know how important sexuality, connection and intimacy is to our quality of life, our resilience and coping. What could be more important!

'Sex' in this book refers to the act, or the activity you engage in with yourself and/others, and is one of the most diverse and most adaptable functional activities I can think of. Yet today, it's still one of the most under-addressed topics in clinical settings. This is something I aim to change.

I also want us all to be on the same page in how we see 'sex' itself which is more than just orgasms and genital play, it's so much more. During cancer treatments and other life-altering events, you might need to temporarily let go of traditional forms of touch/sex. We can become excited, aroused, release pleasure hormones in our body from so many different ways. There are erogenous zones all over our bodies such as our inner thighs, breasts, nipples, under the armpits, the neck, earlobes, feet and many more depending on your body. Orgasms, engorgement, ejaculation, becoming 'hard' or 'wet', these don't need to be your goal, but can also be experienced in more than one way. Pleasure, enjoyment, arousal, excitation and connection, that is where the fun can also be. Pleasure is pleasurable and our whole body can be pleasured!

Desire vs arousal

Desire (the wanting) I use interchangeably with libido. Desire/libido are the experience of *wanting* sex and pleasure. Desire has many words that can be used, such as lust, sex-drive, and essentially all refer to that *want* we have.

Arousal is the way our body responds when it's in pleasure, the changes in our body that show us we are in fact, enjoying and excited. Things like increased sensitivity, maybe we become wet, maybe we become hard, our heart rate increases, we breathe heavier and more.

Simply put, libido = wanting, and arousal = enjoying.

Treatments can affect our arousal as well as our libido and knowing the difference between these can be very helpful.

The magical word, intimacy

Disconnection from yourself and others is a common side-effect of cancer treatments for so many. You're not alone in this and here I introduce you to the magical word 'intimacy'. Imagine that you having sex or being intimate again with yourself, a date or a partner/s, is the goal or the prize. That prize is on the other side of a river, and to get to it, you need to build a bridge. How can you do that? Through intimacy, through touch and the other magical word *affection*.

I've heard many times from clients and people in my support group "we don't even touch each other anymore". Not only has sex gone, but so has the *intimacy*, and are we really going to want sex without that connection?

Intimacy and affection are small giants. Tiny little things that can mean the world, and build that bridge of connection. Things like hand-holding, a good-night kiss, a good morning hug, your arm around your partner in the kitchen, cuddling on the couch, touch for the sake of touch (not as a way to 'get somewhere'), massage swaps, maybe a cheeky butt-squeeze and grin, and the big one, WORDS OF LOVE.

When you want some touch or love? Here's a few ways to ask, without that pressure of it needing to lead to sex:

How to say it out loud.

- "Hey, I'd like to be closer to you, how about a cuddle?"
- "Can we snuggle together on the couch while watching this film?"
- "You up for some hand-holding while we walk to the shop?"
- "I'm loving you right now, thought I'd share."
- "You up for some underwear-on cuddling while we fall asleep? I miss connecting with you."
- "I'd love some touch/to touch your body, would you like a massage?"
- "I'm not wanting this to lead to sex, but some kisses and cuddles would be lovely if you're feeling like some connection?"
- "I'm checking you out right now, just wanted to share."

- "I'm running a bath to relax and wind-down from the day, would you like to join me for some down-time?"

Small giant steps towards that prize.

2.   CONNECTION

When people hear the word 'connection', some assume it means something to do with sex. Well, that is not necessarily always the case as there are so many different types of meaningful connection in our lives, which I'll discuss here.

Connection could be the sharing of intimacy through affection with another, or with yourself. It can make you warm, bring you closer to someone, provide feelings of value and being loved. A hug from a friend, a hand-hold from a family member, even a simple smile from a stranger. Connection, belonging, it all can have a positive impact on us.

Have you heard of the hormone oxytocin? It's referred to as the 'cuddle hormone'. Not only is this hormone released in the body during arousal, but softer, slower forms of touch, such as hand holding or cuddles (just to name a few) can also produce this pleasure hormone. This proves that you can still feel connected, even from the simplest forms of touch such as a hug or soft kiss on the cheek, and why intimacy is so important for our general wellbeing.

There will be relationships and connections in your life that become distant after a diagnosis and there are many reasons for this. Some relationships will struggle, some will fail, some simply might not understand how unwell you are and others might leave or pull away. I lost people during my treatments; people very close to me. I was not coping at all; I was struggling while trying to survive and put walls around me. It's sad, but not an uncommon story. Remember, one of the most difficult things you can experience during treatment is the challenge of putting yourself first. You're fighting for your life, you must. It's how you will manage to face each day. It's how you will survive. Know that other relationships can get stronger, deeper, more loving and connected, and you may even end up with stronger supports and connections around you than before.

Why connecting is essential
I want to share a 'light bulb' moment I had during chemotherapy, one that helped me change a lot about the way I connected to those around me.

I was 4 months into chemotherapy and had just switched to having chemo weekly. It was a sweltering 38-

degree Australian summer night and I walked out of a poetry reading with a friend, to go home. While walking, he hooked his arm through mine, as a sign of affection and connection. When his arm linked through mine, I noticed that I jumped at the touch. Noticing my reaction and how much I had been startled at the contact, it dawned on me. How long had it been since I had been touched in a way that was not medical, hurried and detached? Three weeks? Maybe four? I was so used to the non-intimate hands of nurses, oncologists, surgeons etc. who were not aggressive, but let's say, purposefully unaffectionate in their touch. It was a shock to receive this wonderful soft, intimate connection of an arm slipping through mine. I realised I had become an object of analysis and procedure, and was no longer one of affection. It was shocking to me and it also saddened me.

That was the moment I realised I was losing connection, that was the moment I saw I was becoming detached and I needed to be more vocal. The people around me were being respectful and careful not to touch me, due to how unwell I was. I loved everyone's respectful approach and care towards me as I was very, very sick. I'm grateful for their care, but I realised they also needed guidance from me, to know what was okay and when.

Realising the only touch I had been receiving was medical, which I would switch off to and detach myself from, was one of those 'ahaaa' moments. I had realised how disconnected I had become to my body and that I needed to make the first move and communicate. So, I beg you, educate those around you. Tell your friends they can hold your hand, your family members can put their arm around you, a partner or lover can snuggle with you on the couch. Be their guide for your connection. There are some examples on how to do that further on in this book.

3. COMMUNICATING'S HARD, BUT IMPORTANT

Please don't be down on yourself if you're struggling (whether you're a partner or the person diagnosed). Things are hard, things are different. It's okay, there are workarounds (which I'll get into soon). Ignore external pressures and expectations and focus on yourself and each other. Not only do our bodies and lives change from cancer, so do our roles. From partner to patient, lover to carer, friend to carer etc. You can get through it, together.

Silence is the enemy and can be common when we're finding things difficult. Fear and uncertainty are prevalent during treatments and we can withdraw from each other intentionally or unintentionally. It makes sense that we don't talk about the thing that's hard to talk about!

Fear of dating, meeting new people, of hurting a partner, not knowing how their/your new body works or not wanting to cause pain can all be reasons someone withdraws. Plus, your partner/loved one has seen you go through one of the hardest things of your life, be more unwell than ever, it's scary stuff. For reasons above and more, not knowing how to interact and pulling away is common.

For the people with the diagnosis, understanding what is happening in our body and communicating that? That can feel impossible. Either way, humans have not evolved to read minds, so you'll need to break the silence and share what's happening. So often, the concerns we have in our minds seem a lot bigger when they stay in our minds. Talking is key.

And while we're at it, please don't compare yourself to anyone else or any other relationships. It's the fastest way to unhappiness at any level and that includes comparing yourself to yourself, the 'pre-cancer you'. I call myself 'Tess BC' (BC = before cancer) when I'm in that loop. I often think of my pre-cancer body and mind, how I used to have less pain, more energy, body parts that used to be there, how I could remember things and focus on tasks, so you're not alone in this. I constantly remind myself, comparisons to others or the way things used to be won't change anything. It's such an easy pattern to fall into. I'm sorry to be so blunt as it's hard not to think about what has changed and how things used to be, but please try to think ahead. Cancer is different for everyone and every relationship is different.

There are millions of us fighting cancer, with suffering sexuality. It can be scary, but you don't have to do this alone.

Who to ask and how to ask

Communication with your loved ones isn't the only thing that's essential, but also communication with your treating team. Knowing who to ask about sexuality, positioning, care & *safety* is something most of us don't know.

<u>Here's a general summary.</u>

Gynaecologists work with people who have a vulva and/or vagina. Urologists work with those who have a penis. Gastroenterologists and colorectal surgeons work with the digestive system including bowel cancers. Haematologists work with blood and lymphatic cancers. You will also have medical professionals relative to your treatments such as a radiation oncologist for radiotherapy treatments, an endocrinologist for hormone treatments and the effects they have on our bodies and sexuality, and your oncologist who oversees your treatments. You will have a surgical team relative to the type of procedure you will be having. Psychiatrists are who to speak with regarding mental health and medications, including which medications have which impacts on your sexuality.

All of these people plus your nurses, your doctor or GP (general practitioner if you're in Australia) are all trained to answer your questions.

There are also people like me (OTs) who focus on sexuality, there's pelvic floor physiotherapists and OTs, there are sexologists and sex counsellors as well. You will need to ask; you will need to be your own advocate for your sexuality. But don't worry, if they're not sure how to best answer your question, they will find someone who is. Your care is their priority.

I hear you saying "sure Tess, it's easy to tell us to ask medical professionals questions, but *how* do you ask the questions?" The first step (asking) is the hardest…. But you can do it, I've got your back!

How to say it out loud.

- "What are the precautions I need to take regarding sexual activities during this treatment?"
- "Do I need to avoid sex or do specific things safety-wise? If so, when and for how long?"
- "What do I and my partner/s need to know or do

regarding intimate activities?"

- "I'd like to ask a few questions about sex and intimacy during my treatment. Is there a more private space we could go to?"

- "Is there someone I can speak with, who can answer questions about sex during and after treatment?"

- "We/I would like to discuss intimacy during/after treatment. Can we organise a time? And with who?"

- "I'm experiencing some pain with my (insert issue here). Who is the best person to speak to?"

- "How will this treatment affect me/us intimately?"

- "How long after surgery should we wait until it's okay to have sex again? And are there any positions or movements we should avoid?"

- "I'm not sure how to ask this, but I have some questions of a more private nature, who can I speak with about that?"

- "I'm experiencing pain and it's impacting my private life, who can I speak with about this?"

- "Do I need to avoid sex or do specific things safety-wise during this treatment? If so, when and for how long after the infusion/procedure?"

If a healthcare professional isn't sure or cannot answer your question?

- "Thanks for letting me know, can you please ask someone who might be able to answer?"

- "Okay, can you please tell me who I can ask?"

4.   MANAGING PAIN

Pain is extremely complex and has many forms, be it chronic, neurological, musculoskeletal and more. This section is in reference to people experiencing pain from treatments and is very general. Your treating team is there to help you with your pain, specific to your body and medical history. For people who have pre-existing neurological conditions, past injury, chronic illness, trauma or are living with disability, pain may have been a part of your life well before treatments. If you're someone experiencing pain from treatments and have pre-existing conditions, please chat to your treating team. In particular, your oncologist, doctor, physiotherapist or OT who may be able to connect you with a pain clinic.

Regarding pain experienced from treatments, side effects can persist and our body can take time to heal. We may experience pain from surgeries, radiotherapy, bone pain from endocrine treatments, nerve pain from chemo and more, in many different ways.

You know the saying "no pain, no gain?" We're often given the message that if we want to make progress that it's going to have to hurt. While this can be true at the gym (depending on how you work out), this concept doesn't belong in sex and intimacy.

I once heard a sexuality educator say "no pain, *no pain*" and I instantly loved it. Sex shouldn't ever be painful. Pain is our body's alarm system to let us know something isn't quite right, it's useful information. If you push through it, it won't be pleasurable and it's not going to contribute to you wanting to go back for more. In fact, it could have the opposite effect and put you off. Sex and intimate touch should *never* cause pain, regardless if you have an illness or not. Whatever your age, gender, health status, orientation or pleasures, you should never experience pain during sex and if you do, you should stop. Experiencing painful anal or vaginal penetration (take a look at the mini-book 'A Better Normal for Vaginal Dryness & Pain' for help), or genital pain can be frustrating, but know that it's common and is often overcome. If it's painful or sore and you don't stop, it could cause even more damage. Remember, 'no pain, *no pain'*. Be gentle with yourself, there are plenty of ways to connect.

Planning around pain.

I found that it was best to plan to have connection when I

felt the most well, and was experiencing the least pain during my days and weeks. Try tracking your pain with a calendar or diary, throughout the days and weeks, even with just a simple 0-10 number system you can note in your phone calendar or maybe a paper diary. The aim is to be able to identify patterns, to find times when pain is lower or is absent, or maybe when your painkillers take best effect so you can plan for connection around those times. My pain was very unpredictable in its varied forms, however by keeping a record and flicking through my notes, I did find patterns which enabled me to predict when I would be experiencing less pain in my routine. After exercise was when my pain was lower, also, during chemo, I was able to predict the days when my migraines would start and end. Seeing I would be very unwell for 8-10 days helped me schedule something before I was 'clocking off' into what I then called my 'migraine-holes'. It also gave me something to look forward to after those pain-episodes, a lovely lunch with a friend, a partner coming over or some massage swaps after my migraines subsided. I needed those little lights at the end of each pain-tunnel.

<u>Alternatives.</u>

From tracking your pain in a diary, you may notice a few themes, such as things that can cause a flare-up or more pain. Common things are physically exerting activities like housework, buying groceries, or not having rest breaks throughout the day. Just like I discuss in the mini-book 'A Better Normal for Fatigue', I suggest you break up your daily activities with restful tasks in between. Spacing out the tasks which take a toll on your body, so you can rest in between or time them around your pain meds can be a game changer.

Below is an example of what a client and I came up with, to spread out their demanding tasks. They were self-employed and of course, your life will be completely different to this. But I hope it gives you an idea of ways to break up activities and have rest breaks. Even if it's only one or two days of the week this type of scheduling is possible, or switching around only a few daily tasks in your week, it's better than nothing. Anything is better than nothing!

Time of day	Activity	Energy level
0800	Shower & dress	Uses energy
0830	Breakfast, have meds, watch the news (seated)	Resting
0900	Computer work	Uses energy
1000	See a client	Uses energy
1115	Rest in chair, while doing computer admin on laptop	Resting
1200	Make & eat lunch	Uses energy
1245	Phone a friend/family, lying down/seated in chair	Resting

1300	Go to an appointment/see another client	Uses energy
1430	Light exercise	Creates energy
1500	Get groceries delivered, continue work/see a client	Uses energy
1730	Solo-pleasure/partnered-pleasure time & rest	Can create energy!
1830	Dinner (cook/get delivered)	Uses energy
1930	Rest & digest, & get couch snuggly	Resting

2100	Tidy up kitchen, maybe prep breakfast for tomorrow?	Uses energy
2130	Go to bed, maybe more rest: reading/TV.	Resting

You can also find alternatives, shortcuts and life-hacks depending on what you find causes you pain. If vacuuming causes a flare-up, can you by yourself or a friend gift you a robo-vac? If buying and carrying groceries is too much, can you get them delivered or order online? If standing to cook increases pain, can you sit on a stool in the kitchen while chopping veggies and stirring? Or do a bulk cook on Sundays so you can reheat meals during the week? Can a friend come over and help you with that? Maybe sitting at a desk for too long causes pain, so set an alarm every 30-40 minutes so you can regularly stretch and move your body. These may seem small, but finding these little life-shortcuts can offer relief and reduce flare-ups to give you more capacity for the good things, like intimacy and connection.

Relaxation.

Anticipation, anxiety and stress around intimacy can cause our muscles to become tense and this can increase or contribute to pain. Try to relax. Go slowly. Explore your body alone, use touch, slowly gauge your body and its responses. If you're planning sex, have a nice bath beforehand or warm up with a massage first. It's better to take more time and experience more enjoyment, than to push yourself and have a shorter, less enjoyable time. Plus, when we're not enjoying something or 'forcing' ourselves, our body tenses up and can cause more discomfort. This is not only a way to cause more pain, but also a way to lower your libido, as your brain will associate sex as painful, an obligation and something that is not enjoyable.

Warmth.

Joint and muscle pain can cause discomfort and really got in the way of my wanting to connect with those around me. I found that warmth really helped me. Having a warm shower or bath can help relax your muscles and ease joint pain as it creates blood flow. Just make sure you always have water within arm's reach, as dehydration can exacerbate pain! If you want to engage in self/solo-sex, pleasuring yourself in the bath is ideal if you can get comfortable. Your body is warm and relaxed, two key elements that help with experiencing pleasure.

Don't have a bath? Get your hands on an 'electric throw', a blanket that is heated and you can lie on it or under it during intimate activities. Or warm the bed in advance with an electric blanket or hot water bottle. With a little planning and prep, things can be easier.

Experiment with positions.
If you have pain, alternative positions can be explored or using cushions to support joints or change pelvic angles. Where there is a will, there is usually a way! Keep a sense of humour and exploration about it and know that what worked last time might not work the next time. Refer to the 'sexual positions' section coming up in this book for specific examples.

Go slow and communicate.
It's essential when you're exploring ways to engage intimately and you have any type of pain, to go slowly and communicate. Stop any activity that doesn't feel right. It could be that you're not aroused enough yet, you may need

to avoid certain movements for a while after surgery or it might be that you need to speak with a doctor to determine what is causing the pain and how to treat it. It's okay, there are options and it's worth remembering it may not be permanent.

It isn't spontaneous, but having a comfortable, more pleasurable connection is much more important than having a surprising one. And remember, talk to your medical treating team.

It's worth noting here, that the happy chemicals pleasure, arousal and orgasms release in our body can also relieve pain. I have many clients with chronic illness and disability who use pleasure as pain relief, so they can have moments in their life pain free. Just one more reason why pleasure is so healthy for us!

For those curious as to why I've left out the topic of vaginal pain and dryness out of this section, don't worry. It's such an important and complex topic it has its own mini-book in this series, so take a look at 'A Better Normal for Vaginal Dryness & Pain' for solutions to help vulvovaginal pain, atrophy, painful penetration and all about lubricants and internal moisturisers that help.

5. CHANGES IN SENSATION

I've been speaking quite generally about how we can rehabilitate our desire and strengthen our pleasure pathways, but I'm going to get a little more specific in this section. In particular, the loss of sensation and erogenous zones through treatments, pain and medications, and how losing sensation doesn't necessarily mean losing your sexuality.

I had a breast removed and reconstructed from my lower back tissue nearly two years ago and as I type this, still have no nipple. The breast is firm, a different shape, points in a different direction, feels colder to the touch (could be in my mind) and has zero sensation (not in my mind). I still experience pain on multiple parts of my body, on my skin and also deep within my body structures, completely changing my sensation and sense of touch/pleasure. Initially, I was in my head about it, feeling self-conscious, embarrassed and anxious (especially the one nipple missing part). Losing sensation and pleasure is still hard for me. I miss it; I've lost a piece of my sexuality and I hear this from so many others I support, in reference to not only breasts, but other body parts that have been removed or lost sensation from pain and treatments.

The amazing thing about the human body is that we can create *new* erogenous zones! Remember, our sex and pleasure are what's between our ears and not our legs.

You can 'create' and 'recreate' highly pleasurable erogenous zones all over (and in) your body, with slow soft touch and being present to how good it feels. In particular, if you're feeling numbness and loss of sensation on or in your genitals, repeated touch and in particular massage can 100% help you regain your sensation and pleasure (refer to the 'Vulva Pleasure Masterclass' and 'Penis Pleasure Masterclass' information in the 'resources' section). If you have loss of sensation due to permanent nerve damage or removal, over time, you can have such amazing pleasure from other areas of your body (neck/inner thighs/ears/lips/belly/lower back etc.). How is this done?

Being intimate, focussing on *slow touch* while being curious can start the rewiring process. It's how we create new erogenous zones and enhance pleasure/sensation that may already be there, but just isn't very strong. If you're wanting to recover sensation and pleasure on/in your genitals, I can't recommend soft penis massage and vulva massage highly enough. Even just twice a week has great outcomes over time. If you're experience hypersensitivity on your genitals (overwhelming and overly intense sensations), this can also be neurologically rewired to become less sensitive, less overwhelming and more pleasurable (again, refer to the 'Vulva Pleasure Masterclass' and 'Penis Pleasure Masterclass' information in the 'resources' section).

If you're wanting to recover and improve sensation on your body, take turns in giving and receiving soft slow touch with a blindfold on, offer yourself soft slow touch when you wake up in the morning for 5 minutes each day or if you need extra support and guidance, my online 'connection & cancer' course (detailed in the 'resources' section). Your inner thighs can be just as erotic as say, your breasts once were with touch.

I've used the same techniques to help people post-stroke regain sensation on their arms, when working in neurological rehabilitation. With a little repetition and attention, you can enhance your pleasure and sensitivity too. Neurological change doesn't happen overnight, but over time it can and does happen.

Remember, pleasure is still pleasurable, even if it's somewhere else on your fabulous body.

In the meantime, brain-chatter from things like self-consciousness, anxiety or stress can be the barrier to enjoying touch on your body and also that rewiring process. If you're getting intimate and feeling self-conscious about your body, pop a little lacy number on, or an item of clothing that's a lovely, sensual material. Something that *feels* nice and helps reduce the anxiety. This will help get your head back into the experience.

Remember, it's okay to get sexy while wearing clothing. Or try some positions that aren't so full-frontal to help you relax and enjoy. The key to enhancing your pleasure, to strengthening those sensory and pleasure pathways is to be present, and we can't do that when we're in our heads.

I also want to note that I have a sense of loss. Please allow yourself time to grieve, process and share how you're feeling. None of this is easy, but the loss of sensation on an area of your body doesn't have to mean the loss of your sex or your pleasure all together.

Just like everything else in cancer, it's a process and can take time, but speaking from personal experience as someone who has rehabilitated themselves through these touch and massage practices, it's well worth it.

6.   COMMUNICATING ABOUT SEX

I've mentioned that you will need to be your own sexual advocate and have given many samples for how to ask questions, but it really is so important you do ask them. I'm not just referring to your treating team, but to those around you that you're intimate with. It can seem daunting, which is why I've been littering this book with specific communication examples.

Why you should ask your health care team?

I'm continually asking you to speak up to your treating team, because if you wait for someone to bring it up, it may not happen. Through an almost complete lack of healthcare professionals initiating a conversation on this topic, I learned that I needed to take the initiative myself to ask the questions. Given how important the topic of intimacy, relationships, sexuality and well-being is, don't be shy - always ask, and if you need to, persist. Medical staff may not voluntarily bring it up, but I've found they are often very well-informed once I ask and are more than happy to have those conversations.

I once asked a nurse while I was in the chemo-chair for

advice regarding the ulcers I had on my outer labia. The response I got was calm and not shaming at all, she said she would "ask around" and walked off. She didn't return for over half an hour, so of course I thought she might have been embarrassed and was avoiding the topic, and due to that, I was reluctant to bring it up again. When she eventually returned and didn't mention it, I plucked up some courage and asked her again. The nurse apologised immediately and explained that there was a medical emergency in the next room and it had slipped her mind. She went out to ask the person she was originally going to ask, came back quickly with information, I wrote down the recommendation for a topical cream and everything was fine.

I'm so glad I persisted because my assumption was wrong. The nurse was perfectly happy to discuss it with me, she was just preoccupied with something else. This is a perfect example of how you will need to advocate for yourself and for information about sexuality in clinical settings. Sometimes it's not a priority, but most of the time the staff are so very busy, working tirelessly and these things take a backseat. Another thing that was a pleasant surprise was that the nurses, surgeons, radiologists and pharmacists I spoke to didn't blink an eye when I asked them sexuality-based questions. And they were more than happy to contact the relevant medical professional to answer any questions when they weren't sure what recommendations to give. Medical professionals are trained to talk about bodies, bodily functions and intimate things as part of their job, so, be confident that all you need is to pluck up the courage to ask.

If you do come across a health professional who is uncomfortable when you ask a question or bring up the topic, my suggestion is not to take this personally and just ask someone else, or ask that person who else you could speak with. We've all been brought up with shame around sex and for some healthcare professionals, despite their values and training, might still feel embarrassed. This doesn't have anything to do with you, so please don't take it as a reason to not ask others. You'll find the people around you who are particularly helpful and forthcoming with assistance. I recommend writing their name down so you can focus on directing any questions to them.

Communicating with your partners

Pop-quiz, what am I?

We're not supposed to talk about it, you can't have too much of it, you can't have too little of it, it's used in nearly all marketing to sell but it's never presented accurately in the media, it's a part of human life, social media platforms shut you down for talking about it, people who are different, unwell, older, living with disability, are of different cultures and ethnicities are assumed to not have it or to want it, we receive no education on it yet we're supposed to magically be good at it and we're supposed to always want it....... Yup. That'd be sex.

You may feel from reading the above that you can't win, and sure, our culture doesn't exactly embrace open communication regarding sexuality, but reading this book is how you will learn.

In my experience as a sexuality educator (as well as from my own life), people who are able to talk between themselves about sex more openly, have much better sex. Why, you ask? Because communicating about how you're feeling and what you might enjoy, allows you to engage comfortably and pleasurably. It can also reduce feeling like you're forcing yourself, forcing someone else, or causing any possible harm. It's okay if things have changed, our bodies and pleasure always will. If we can learn how to communicate about what we do or don't want, things will be better. Remember, hand holding, eye contact, cuddles, snuggles on the couch, foot/body/hand massage, genital massage, oral genital play, assisting/giving masturbation, self-touch together, watching pornography together or reading erotic literature together, all of these things are sex and all of them are connective.

I'm going to share a story of someone who wrote about their experience of sex after having their penis removed due to cancer. Post-surgery, he and his wife still have regular sex and are even more satisfied with the quality of their intimacy than before. He shared that before cancer he would ejaculate every time they had sex, which would last around 15 minutes. Now, he has orgasms from his nipples, thighs and scrotum being touched (how amazing is the neuroplasticity of pleasure!). He also now offers his wife many more orgasms and their sex lasts on average an hour. He refers to it as more "quality". They communicate more, explore each other's bodies more and pleasure each other more. A changed body doesn't necessarily mean worse sex or the end of it all together, change can have its rewards.

7. SEXUAL POSITIONS, TECHNIQUES & TOOLS

Sex as a functional activity is extremely adaptable, with so many possible positions we can put our bodies in and so many adaptations to suit our needs. Here, I offer some suggestions and ways to alter the positions of your body to get around some of the trickier side-effects of treatments.

Explore, experiment, but make sure you do it from a place of communication and curiosity. You all want to be comfortable and, most importantly, safe, so have a chat beforehand with your lover. Treat it like a brainstorm, note what parts of your body are sore or might need support and figure out how to work around them comfortably and safely. It mightn't seem 'sexy' at first, but these conversations will get easier, and it will make things *much* better. And remember, if it's good, you'll want it more.

It's important to note, bodies are complicated and what might work one day, might not the next. It's okay, it's normal, but you need to communicate how you're doing during and after sex. Telling your lover that you're needing to change position because the sheet is rubbing on your chemo rash, or that your muscles are starting to get tired, that you need to slow down due to a bit of nausea, or perhaps a drain tube is getting bumped, is important for both of your enjoyment. Comments like this, are you being great at sex. Make the adjustments you need, see if everyone is doing okay, keep going if you're all comfortable and check in after.

If you want to stop, then stop. Remember, don't force it, don't put up with pain, self-pleasure is always there for a partner if someone wants to continue. Hey, if you stop sex as it's a bit too difficult or is no longer pleasurable and your lover wants to continue pleasure through touching themselves? Offer them a hand!

Key positional tricks.

- The more still and supported you are, the less energy you use.
- Having your chest exposed (not against something or someone) can make it easier to breathe.
- Sitting up, and being still is great for people using oxygen and for nausea.
- Having your chest open and staying upright can be more comfortable if you're experiencing acid reflux.
- A pillow/cushion between the knees separates the

thighs and prevents them rubbing together if you have sensitive skin there or a catheter taped to your inner thigh.

- If you're standing up and playing with someone lying on a bed/chair, whether they're on their front or back, you can put some pillows underneath them to raise their pelvis to match the height of yours. This avoids you needing to bend/squat down, which could be tiring or cause joint pain. This is also a great tip if you're playing with or penetrating an anus.

- Empty your stoma pouch/urine collection device before sex and while you're getting used to it. Try positions that leave space around that area such as standing, sitting, lying on your side, being behind someone, or on top of someone.

- If you have a catheter, stoma or drain-tube, communication is key. Chat, brainstorm, explore, you'll be fine!

- If you have tubes or surgery sites, don't lie on them, use cushions to protect them and lie on your other side (your 'unaffected' side) to avoid pushing/putting weight on them.

- Standing or sitting in a corner has more stability than leaning against a flat wall.

- If you're having sex and are using a manual wheelchair? Double check the breaks are on!

- With any wheelchair play, pop the armrests up/take them off if able, it frees up a *lot* of space.

- For wheelchairs that have a tilt-in-space function, this can be great for in-chair partner play!

- If you're uncomfortable deep inside? Use an 'Ohnut' to reduce the depth of penetration.

- Sore joints? Have a bath beforehand or a warm shower and get straight into a warm cosy bed.

- A pillow under your hips raises the pelvis, allowing easier access to the genitals/anus and also supports the lower back.

- A pillow between the thighs can be wonderful for hip & knee joint pain.

- If you find a good position, but it's hard to hold yourself in it? Prop yourself up with cushions or pillows.

- Concerns about continence if you get excited? Having sex in the shower rinses away any urine or faeces that might come out. Avoid using plastic bed sheets as they don't absorb anything and can create more mess. You can pop a towel down on the bed, plus there are great absorbent mats designed for children that wet the bed. I have a 'Squirt Blanket' from Yoni Pleasure Palace, it's machine washable and it's the best.

- Use lubricants, always and forever.
- Get comfy, put cushions under any knees or bums if you're on the ground.
- Lastly, and most importantly, communicate before, during and after about how you're doing.

How to say it out loud.

- "Can we please pause for a second? I just need to re-adjust these cushions, thanks!"
- "I'd love to keep going, but we may need to brainstorm a new position as I'm a bit sore/tired/out of breath…"
- "I'm really loving this, could we slow down a bit? I'm starting to ache a bit."
- "This is so great, but I'm having a hot flush, can we sit up so I'm not in so much contact with the bed?"
- "I'm really enjoying this; I just need to top up the

lube."

- "It's wonderful to connect with you, but I'm starting to feel a little dry, can you pass the lube please?"
- "Pause, lube top-up!"
- "I'm feeling some discomfort/changes in my erection, how do you feel about some pleasuring with my hands?"
- "I may need to stop; would you like to continue with self-pleasure? Would you like me to touch your body while you pleasure yourself?"
- "Can we please pause? I'm feeling a bit odd and need a moment, thank you."
- "I don't want to keep going as we are, but really want to continue being intimate with you. Is there some form of different touch or pleasure you might enjoy that I can offer you?"
- "How could you/we enjoy this more?"
- "Is there a speed or pressure of touch that you might enjoy more?"
- "How could this be even better for both of us?"
- "I just wanted to check in, are you comfortable?"
- "Please let me know if you need to change positions

at any time."

- "Please call out for more lube if/when you need, it's within arm's reach."
- "I'm loving connecting with you, I just want to make sure you're comfortable?"
- "I know I'm not moving much, but I'm really enjoying this and I'd like to keep going."

Communicating after intimacy (aftercare).

- "Thank you so much, that was wonderful. Is there anything you need or would like in this moment?"
- "Can we please cuddle for a while? I'd like to stay connected with you for a bit longer."
- "I'd love to know what you enjoyed about that experience, and I'll share the same."
- "I'd love to know if there was anything you might like to do differently next time, or explore more, and I'll share the same."
- "Can we lie here together while I catch my breath?"
- "This has brought up a few emotions, I'm okay, but chatting for a short while would be lovely."

8.   HAEMORRHOIDS AND ANAL FISSURES

Warning, Tess over-share coming! My cancer treatment side-effects and impacts were endless. From my first type of chemotherapy, the oh-so appropriately nicknamed 'red devil' I experienced severe constipation, causing haemorrhoids and anal fissures. Then, when I switched to the weekly "not-so-shit" chemo as my oncologist called it, I had chronic diarrhoea - causing more haemorrhoids. And just when I thought it couldn't get any worse, with that new chemo I also experienced constant sneezing fits. Let's think about that for a second. Diarrhoea and sneezing...it was *almost* comical. Anal health and care are a part of my daily routine, not only so I can go to the toilet without crying, but so I can also access pleasure.

There are many topical creams available to treat haemorrhoids, ask your doctor/GP, pharmacist or oncologist what they recommend. A warm, Epsom salt bath can soothe haemorrhoid pain and also relax the sphincters and surrounding muscles. Generally, avoid any anal play until your pain eases and then, please use lubricants. Lubricants are an anuses best friend. If you're using condoms, you have two choices: the regular external condom, AKA the 'male condom' that rolls onto toys and penises, and the internal condom AKA the 'female condom' that can fit inside the anus (and vagina's). Not many folks have heard of the internal condom, but they're available from some chemists, online sex stores and from STI clinics. They're also useful for smaller penises or ones that aren't as hard, and they also offer a different sensation to a standard condom. No matter what you're using, remember that nothing should be inserted anally (even a fingertip) without lubricant.

There are also some anal exercises you can do, to strengthen the sphincters and increase blood flow to the area, which can have positive impacts (I noticed less pain within a day doing this). This may seem strange, but the anal sphincters are connected to our pelvic floor muscles and if they are healthy, able to relax and contract? Not only may pain improve, but also blood flow can increase, which influences healing, arousal and pleasure.

A few exercises are:

1. As you breathe in, clench your anus shut. As you breathe out, relax it (or the opposite way if that

feels more right for you). The release is just as (if not more) important than the clench. The release is the motion that allows blood flow to access the tissues.

2. As you breathe in, clench your anal sphincter about half-way, pause, then clench all the way as hard as you can. Like a two-step clench on the inhale. And then relax on your exhale.

3. Clenching and release your anal sphincter with breath, but much faster.

Do these a few hundred times a day (I'm quite serious) and you may experience improvements such as less pain or going to the toilet easier. To make sure you remember to do it, you could remind yourself to do these exercises when you do a certain daily activity, such as every time you open the fridge, do twenty. Or do 30 when you sit down for a coffee, are stopped at a traffic light or when you go to bed.

If you have had any type of bowel, rectal or pelvic surgery, please have a discussion with your surgeon / oncologist / doctor / pelvic floor physiotherapist before you start doing any exercises. Pelvic floor physiotherapists are incredible for regaining strength in this area.

If you experience pain when doing any pelvic floor/anal strengthening exercises, stop doing them immediately and speak with your treating team. And of course, if you're in pain and topical ointments are not helping, see a doctor.

9.   TIPS FOR LOVED ONES

Seeing a loved one go through cancer is tough, and so can knowing what to say or how to act. Whether you're a carer, friend, family member or partner, there are ways to offer connection without overstepping a line. And don't worry, we won't break!

Yes, caution is (very) necessary and the medical team must tell you about all of the risks involved in all treatments. People in pain, undergoing chemo, surgeries, radiotherapy, we can be seen as easily hurt, fragile or dangerous, and rightly so. There are many side-effects of treatments, some of them are mental and some of them are physical. However, let's remember this: connection is always important, and even if someone's body and mind are changing, there are still ways to be there with someone.

It can understandably be hard to know what to do. It's also normal, when seeing a loved one be so unwell, to want to avoid causing any other harm and through that, create physical distance. That might look like reducing touch and physical contact, or even like possible avoidance. If you're a partner, lover, friend or carer of someone during treatment, I implore you, I beg you, to offer them touch. Treatment is damaging and also detaching. We need the treatment, yes, but we also need care, to feel connected to ourselves and to those around us. Don't be afraid of us, be cautious and curious with us. Think of it as getting into 'ask first' mode.

For simple touch, a peck on the lips or cheek? It's okay! We are not radioactive, we won't give you cancer and we won't break, if we all just take a little care. How do we know what to do or what not to do? We ask.

How to say it out loud.
- "Would you like me to take your hand?"
- "Is there any way you might like some loving/comforting touch right now?"
- "Would you like a hug?"
- "I'd love a cuddle; how does that sound to you?"
- "I'd love to connect with you, are there any sore spots I should avoid if I went in for a cuddle?"
- "I'd love to connect with you right now, is there a form of touch you would like?" (Arm around the shoulder, hand holding, hug from behind, foot massage and more.)
- "I love you and want to offer you affection, is there anything that would comfort you at the moment?"

- "I miss you, but I'm worried I'll hurt you if I squeeze you too hard. Is there a way I can snuggle into you?"
- "I'm wanting to show you love and affection, such as a kiss on the lips or cheek, how do you feel about that?"
- "I'm checking you out right now, fancy a kiss?"

If you're being made an offer of connection and it's not a good time? I offer some examples shortly on ways to navigate that, however a simple, "thank you, but I'm not quite up for it at the moment" is perfect. Even if the person receiving this offer is not up for it right then, you're showing love, care, concern for their well-being and the desire to remain connected. It means the world.

Not in the mood?

Whether you're the person with cancer or the partner of, there will be times when you don't feel like being intimate with others, that is fine, that is normal, that is understandable. There will also be times when you feel like connecting somehow, but aren't sure how. There are lots of places to start: Get in the bath and relax or wrap yourself in blankets with a hot-water bottle, maybe touch your body, snuggle a pet with your favourite film, ask the person you're with to intertwine your legs while you both sit on the couch or lean into their chest. During treatments, you're not going to want intimacy or touch all of the time, so feel free to let loved ones know how you're feeling and speak up in the moments it seems plausible. If you do receive an offer of intimacy and connection and you're not up for it? Remember, that's okay, that's fine, that's normal. But also remember to say thanks for the offer and be kind when you say no thanks, because you want the offers to keep coming!

How to say it out loud.

- "Thank you, that sounds amazing, it's not the best moment, can we see how I'm going later?" (Or tomorrow, or after lunch)
- "Thanks, I'm feeling some pain so for the moment I need to sit still, can we maybe connect later or another day?"
- "I'm really not feeling well, I'd like to sit alone for a while. Thank you so much for offering a cuddle, rain-check?"

- "I'd love to kiss you, but my mouth is a bit sore at the moment, would you like some soft neck touch instead?"
- "I'd love a hug, thank you, could you be careful around my arm? It's a bit sore."
- "I don't think I'm up for a hug right now, would you like to hold my hand?"
- "I'm pretty low on energy at the moment, but something soft and gentle would be lovely, like a snuggle?"
- Or if you're ADHD and ridiculously blunt like me "Thanks for the offer of a kiss, I'm currently trying not to vomit in my mouth, so will need to rain-check" (we both had a giggle at that).

To those undergoing treatments, if you feel your partner/lover/friend is avoiding you, unattracted to you and doesn't want to touch you? They may just be thinking they are protecting you, avoiding potentially hurting you or feel like they're pestering/pressuring you, so are pulling away. Be the one to communicate and offer a connection. Offer to snuggle, offer to touch their back while they're standing next to you, ask for a long hug hello, it guides them, and can lead to further connections. It meant the world to me, having my hand held and legs entwined on the couch with a cup of tea and chats. Simple things like that were so important, and I know is/was to others during treatments.

10. A FUN WAY TO CONNECT

I'll be honest, during my more intense chronic pain periods, sometimes intimacy felt like it was completely off the table. However, the below 'game' was my saviour. I simply love it as it can be super intimate, but also super fun, and totally works around how you're feeling in the moment.

The two-minute game

Life coach Harry Faddis created the 'three-minute game' and I was taught the 'two-minute game' from Roger Butler at Curious Creatures, and it's simply brilliant. This game is suitable for those experiencing treatment and their loved ones, is great when you have no idea how to connect with someone or where to start and is a wonderful way to gently get to know each other's bodies again.

Here's the rules.

- Set a timer or an alarm on your phone for two minutes.

- Pick who goes first, then that person asks for something they would like for 2 minutes (some examples are listed shortly).

- If you all agree, start the timer and give the person

whatever they asked for.

- When the timer goes off, completely stop what you're doing.

- Then it's the next person's turn to ask for something they would like for two minutes.

- If everyone agrees, start the timer and go.

- Once the timer goes off, again, stop what you're doing.

- And repeat.

That's it. Really, that is the game. So simple, yet so effective. You can play it for as long as you like - 10 minutes or an hour, or however long you have energy and are having fun. Time can really fly when playing this game.

Also, this game can be played with anyone, not just someone you're in a relationship with. It could be a friend, family member, carer and doesn't have to be in pairs. There are so many ways to connect, to touch and be touched, which this game can help you discover.

One of the first (out of possibly hundreds) times I played this, I wasn't sure what to ask for. So, of course, I asked for a shoulder massage. Then, that became a slow back scratch. Then full body soft touch and I was amazed at how starting simply and being left wanting more (thanks to that timer) guided me to what I would like next. Asking for what you want can be difficult at first, but this game allows you to develop that skill with practice. Asking for what we want is such an essential skill to have during cancer treatments (and always).

A common question when introducing the two-minute game in workshops is, "what happens if someone asks for something you don't want to do?" Say "no-thank you" with a smile and discuss an alternative (such as touching the chest or back rather than genitals). It's okay. Wait, it's more than okay, it's wonderful to say 'no'. Saying what we don't want is equally (maybe more) important than saying what we do want. The goal is to find that optimal place where everyone is happy giving and receiving.

Here's a few reasons why this game can work for you:
Our genitals aren't always up for being played with, so when it's your two minutes, ask for something that doesn't include them (you have your whole body).

This game can allow connection, even with different levels of libido. Someone might want sexual touch for two minutes and if you're happy to give it, great! Your two minutes could be something that suits your mood such as "tell me your favourite joke using your hand as a puppet". The possibilities are endless and you can ask for exactly what you want, while easily avoiding what you don't want.

Bodies impacted by treatment can change dramatically and unpredictably, be it sensation, arousal, pain, surgical sites etc. This game allows you to relearn how your body works or doesn't work (where those desensitised parts are, where it's sore, where it's pleasurable, how toys or lubes feel).

If you're playing this with a partner and are worried about where things may lead to? Take 'typical' sex off the table for the entire game. You could have a 'no genital contact' rule or even leave your clothes on. Remove the pressure to perform or get aroused. Obligation & expectation are the enemy of arousal, feeling safe and relaxed is its catalyst. Get creative, enjoy yourselves without that pressure. You can enjoy pleasure from soft intimate touch anywhere on the body.

The two-minute game has many communication benefits and can act as a gentle ice breaker. With changed sexuality and changed intimacy (with or without illness), can come distance and avoidance. Talking about sex is not easy, especially when things are different. This game gently offers a way to help navigate those tricky feelings while also acknowledging the elephant in the room. While we're at it, let's erase any feelings of 'being selfish' or 'a taker'. Asking for your neck to be gently kissed for two minutes, or to be told why this person loves you for two minutes, is simply playing the game. It can seem difficult, but remember, you have to ask, it's the rules! Through my work as a sexuality and consent workshop facilitator, I'm always shocked at how many people tell me that they have never asked for what they want before. Practice makes perfect and it does get easier the more you do it.

Here's a list of things you could ask for, for your two minutes:

- Can you please lower the lights, put some relaxing music on that I would like, bring me water and join me on the couch in two minutes?
- Hold my hand and tell me how you're doing for two minutes.
- Massage my (insert body part here) for two minutes.
- Starting at my neck, ever so softly touch my entire body, back to feet over two minutes.
- Tell me about your day through interpretive dance.

- Put on a song and show me your silliest/favourite dance move.

- Make me a cup of tea in two minutes.

- I would like to cuddle for two minutes.

- I would like to offer you a shoulder massage for two minutes (that's still your two minutes, but if you're not up for being touched, you can touch others. It's all about what YOU want).

- Massage my head.

- I would like to stroke your hair with your head in my lap.

- Lightly touch my beautiful bald head for 2 minutes.

- Gently kiss my neck/chest/thighs/back for two minutes.

- Show me how you like to be kissed, for two minutes.

- Kiss my face and tell me things you love about me for two minutes.

- Softly breathe on my entire body, ending with my genitals for two minutes (YUM!).

If you're thinking, "ugh, whatever Tess. Some of us don't know how to just simply know what you want and ask for it." You're right, I hear you. None of us are taught this. This game is a wonderful way to practice and learn this essential bedroom-skill. Be kind to yourself and start slow, you may be quite surprised how natural and fun it can feel after a few rounds!

11.   FOR MY FELLOW RAINBOW-FLAGGERS

For people in the LGBTQIA+ community, medical institutions can be very difficult. I remember sitting in the chemo-chair with my then partner holding my hand. The nurse approached and looked at us holding hands, then looking at her said "oh, isn't that sweet you're such good *friends*". I know the nurse meant well, but it was devaluing to me and my partner. I did not feel like I was seen as a person, nor my partner respected. I also did not have the energy to continually educate everyone around me all day every day and advocate for who I am and for others. It's exhausting and with cancer, I didn't have it in me. So, I withdrew and I became reluctant to share my personal story with most clinicians. This is particularly important for people with cancers such as prostate, testicular, cervix, ovaries or breast (just to name a few), as these cancers are *very* gendered. Due to this people can isolate themselves from the supports that are out there as they may feel unwelcome or unseen. Speaking personally, the 'sisterhood' is very strong in breast cancer and as a non-binary person, was difficult to ignore. I avoided so many (pretty much all) support networks due to this as I did not feel welcome. If you're someone who resonates with this, if you belong to communities that are marginalised, I ask you to reach out. Reach out to that one person on your treating team you can have an honest, non-shaming conversation with. Reach out to the nurse asking for any resources the hospital knows of that are accessible and inclusive. Reach out to a friend, to find a cancer support group near you or online that is gender aware, recognises pronouns, alternative relationship models, and partnerships that are not only heterosexual. They are out there, but you may need help finding them. Feeling safe and supported is everything.

RESOURCES

Because there's limited work on sexuality and cancer and well, actual realistic and accessible sexuality education in general, resources can be hard to find. So, here are some, of varied mediums depending on what suits you best.

The 'A Better Normal' mini-book series

Available globally on Amazon in paperback or eBook format, you can search by author 'Tess Devèze' or by book title.

If you're needing support, practical solutions and guidance on more specific side-effects, or looking for help regarding a specific treatment, the 'A Better Normal' mini-book series covers quite a range.

Books in the 'A Better Normal' mini-book series are:

- 'A Better Normal for **Libido**; Your Guide to Rediscovering Intimacy After Cancer'
- 'A Better Normal for **Vaginal Dryness & Pain**; Your Guide to Rediscovering Intimacy After Cancer'
- 'A Better Normal for **Body Confidence**; Your Guide to Rediscovering Intimacy After Cancer'

- 'A Better Normal for **Chemotherapy**; Your Guide to Rediscovering Intimacy After Cancer'
- 'A Better Normal for **Hormone Therapy**; Your Guide to Rediscovering Intimacy After Cancer'
- 'A Better Normal for **Fatigue**; Your Guide to Rediscovering Intimacy After Cancer'
- 'A Better Normal for **Changes in Erection**; Your Guide to Rediscovering Intimacy After Cancer'
- 'A Better Normal for **Radiotherapy**; Your Guide to Rediscovering Intimacy After Cancer'
- 'A Better Normal for **Pain**; Your Guide to Rediscovering Intimacy After Cancer'

The all-in-one resource, 'A Better Normal; Your Guide to Rediscovering Intimacy After Cancer'

Available globally on Amazon in paperback or eBook, you can search via author 'Tess Devèze' or by book title.

If you liked the information in this book, but feel you need guidance on more, the book 'A Better Normal; Your Guide to Rediscovering Intimacy After Cancer' has all of the information included in the entire mini-book series and more. It's your one stop shop for everything you need to know about sexuality and cancer, in the one book.

Vulva Pleasure Masterclass

(connectable.podia.com/vulva-masterclass)

For anyone with a vulva who is experiencing pain and dryness, or is experiencing loss of sensation, pleasure, arousal and orgasm. This online Masterclass teaches vulva massage, which can be done on yourself or with a partner. Through massage and neurological concepts, things like arousal and pleasure can be recovered while helping heal tissues through increasing blood-flow with massage. This Masterclass is also suitable for people with vaginismus and vulvodynia.

Penis Pleasure Masterclass

(connectable.podia.com/penis-pleasure)

For anyone with a penis who is experiencing changes in erection and orgasm, or is experiencing loss of sensation, function and pleasure. This online Masterclass teaches soft penis massage, which can be done on yourself or with a partner. Through massage and neurological concepts, things like sensation and pleasure can be recovered while helping recover erectile function through increasing blood-flow with massage. This Masterclass is particularly beneficial for people post prostatectomy.

A libido and intimacy recovery program for couples

'Connection & Cancer: Reclaim Your Intimacy & Desire'. (connectable.podia.com/libido-after-cancer)

If you would like personal support through the exact process of *how* to recover your pleasure, intimacy and libido, then this is for you. It's with me online guiding you every step of the way, and is done in the privacy of your own home. Filled with information, fun and practical solutions that I take you through for libido recovery. The people who I've worked with in this program are having life-changing results. It's an absolute honour to guide people to recover what they felt was lost forever.

'ConnectAble Therapies' (connectabletherapies.com)

For consultations and further resources on sex, intimacy & cancer.

Facebook global support group: *'Intimacy and Cancer'*. This group is for any cancer, any gender and is a very supportive space.

Instagram '@connectable_therapies', where I regularly share helpful information.

YouTube Channel on sex, intimacy & cancer: type *"Intimacy and Cancer CHANNEL"* to find it.

If you prefer video formats over reading (as cancer-brain & reading don't go well together), this YouTube Channel is filled with short videos discussing all things sex, intimacy and cancer.

'ConnectAble Courses' (connectable.podia.com)
A site of intimacy and cancer online courses for sexual recovery. Including the Masterclasses, libido recovery program and webinar mentioned here.

Intimacy & Cancer Information Webinar
(connectable.podia.com/webinar-intimacyaftercancer)
A free information webinar discussing the impacts cancer treatments have on intimacy and sexuality. It has a particular focus on libido and how it can be recovered.

Other amazing resources:
'A Touchy Subject' (atouchysubject.com)
For people with prostate cancer or experiencing changes in erection. Victoria Cullen is *the* person to go to, about sexuality and intimacy post a prostate cancer diagnosis. She

also has a YouTube channel and through her website access to free resources and rehabilitation programs.

'The Art of The Hook Up' (artofthehookup.com)

This site from dating expert and communication extraordinaire is by Georgie Wolf. Not cancer specific, but incredibly on-point and with relative information for anyone struggling with the dating scene. She has podcasts, blogs, eBooks and more. She's also a workshop facilitator and a bit of a superstar here in Australia!

'Curious Creatures' (curiouscreatures.biz)

For online workshops and much more education on self-development and sexuality. They provide articles, podcasts and streamable workshops which are all very practical and very accessible. I have the privilege to work for this company, their work is changing lives.

'Bump'n Joystick' (getbumpn.com)

An intimacy aid designed for people with impaired upper limb and fine-motor function. Suitable for all genders and is flexible to varied body shapes. This toy was designed by the global disability and OT community, and it's pretty incredible.

'The Ziggy' (luddi.co)

Another intimacy aid designed for people with limited upper limb and intact fine-motor function. Designed by the disability community and healthcare professionals, this is a multi-purpose vibrator for all genders. It's also able to be used while in a wheelchair, so is a wonderfully accessible item.

Pelvic and sexual health osteopath

For those who live in Melbourne, Australia, we have one of the top pelvic health osteopaths you'll ever find. Dr Andrew Carr from the *'Whole Being Health Collective'* is referred to as *'the body whisperer'* in clinical and sexual health circles. He works with the entire body, however has expertise and clinical focus on pelvic and sexual health. In particular, people experiencing pelvic pain including after treatments, vaginismus, atrophy and is trauma informed.

If you're not located in Melbourne, there are pelvic floor osteopaths, physiotherapists and OTs all over the world. Simply search online "Pelvic floor osteopath/physio/OT (insert the name of your city/town here)". You'll find someone near you.

Support groups in your area

If you search in google "Cancer Support (insert city/town where you live here)", there should be a list of businesses and companies that have programs near you. Some online or in person. They mightn't be sexuality specific, but there is always opportunity for discussions and learning.

ACKNOWLEDGEMENTS

For anyone and everyone out there affected by cancer, this book is for you. There can be so much to consider, to have to endure, to have to keep track of, that many parts of life take a back seat. Thank you for caring about your intimacy and connections during such a time, be it connections with yourself or with others. I hope you're supported and I truly hope there is something in this book for you.

I'm forever grateful to my clients and the thousands I support online who so openly and vulnerably share their struggles, and also their triumphs with me. This book would not exist without you. I'm inspired and amazed by you all, daily.

Thank you, to my partners and carers over the years Rog, Robi and Kane, my family and my global network of friends. There were some very dark places during treatments and you all got me through. To my booby buddies (my breast care nurses) Claire & Monique, you're my angels. Ricky Dick my oncologist - you're simply the best (Tina Turner style!) and to my RADelaidies.

Lastly, to acknowledge the incredible ethics, values and

approaches to sexuality and communication from Roger Butler at Curious Creatures (and their generosity with sharing their content with me), the occupational therapy & sexuality community (yeah OT-siggers!) and the revolutionary perspectives and therapeutic trainings I received from Deej & Uma, at the Institute of Somatic Sexology (ISS).

ABOUT THE AUTHOR

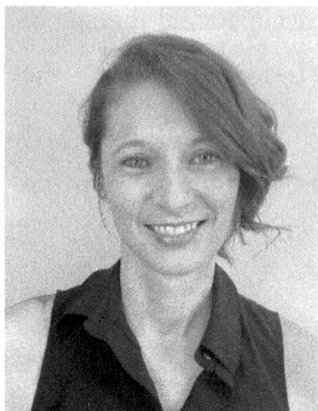

Tess Devèze is an occupational therapist (OT) having completed their bachelor degree in Melbourne Australia, founding ConnectAble Therapies, a community sexuality OT and sexology clinic focussing on sexuality and intimacy for people with neurological conditions, cancer, chronic illness and disability. They have also completed certification and trainings via the Institute of Somatic Sexology. Alongside being a sexuality OT, Tess is also a sexuality educator & workshop facilitator, and has facilitated and educated thousands of people in the topics of communication, consent, sexuality, pleasure and relationship dynamics for nearing a decade. Tess founded the global online initiative 'Intimacy and Cancer', an online support space for people of all cancers and genders to access sexual support.

As a non-binary, queer, disabled person living with cancer, Tess's work is inclusive and advocates for sexual rights for disabled, neurodivergent, gender queer/diverse and LGBTQIA+, communities, which they proudly belong to.

Tess was diagnosed with stage 3 breast cancer at the age of 36 and is still undergoing treatments.

Find them at www.connectabletherapies.com

DID YOU ENJOY THE BOOK?

As an independent author, my work survives through your support. There are so many people affected by cancer, suffering in silence. With each review or word-of-mouth recommendation you make, we can reach the many out there who are struggling and need support.

Please leave a review by visiting where you purchased this book. It's just 1 minute of your time, but could be the thing that helps this reach someone who needs it, someone who needs a better normal too.

Got feedback? Please leave a review! Plus, I'd love to hear from you. You can reach me via email at tess@connectabletherapies.com or via Instagram @connectable_therapies.